HERPES TREATMENT MANUAL

A comprehensive guide on   treatment of herpes for good healthy living

Dr Rowan Theo

Table of Contents

CHAPTER ONE 3

   Herpes 3

CHAPTER TWO 12

   HSV and HIV 12

CHAPTER THREE 21

   What reasons genital sores in ladies? 21

CHAPTER FOUR.......................29

   Molluscum contagiosum 29

THE END..................................40

CHAPTER ONE

Herpes

Herpes effects from contamination with the herpes simplex virus (HSV). It reasons sores or blisters to shape in or across the mouth or genitals, in addition to different signs.

There are kinds of HSV:

• HSV-1 reasons oral herpes, which commonly influences the mouth and surrounding pores and skin.

• HSV-2 reasons genital herpes, that's commonly sexually transmitted.

If someone has an HSV contamination, they'll have it for the relaxation in their life, aleven though a few human beings by no means expand signs. If signs arise, they replicate the form of HSV.

There isn't any remedy for herpes, however remedy can assist control signs and decrease the probability of them ordinary.

round 67% of human beings, globally, have an HSV-1 contamination, and 11% have an HSV-2 contamination.

Symptoms

People who expand signs of herpes might also additionally first revel in tingling, itching, or burning, then word sores or blisters forming across the mouth or genitals.

Symptoms have a tendency to expand 2–20 days after publicity to the virus.

Oral herpes

Oral herpes reasons blisters, occasionally known as fever sores or bloodless sores, to expand in or across the lips and mouth.

Sometimes those blisters shape some place else at the face or at the tongue, and greater hardly

ever on different regions of pores
and skin.

The sores commonly closing 2–
three weeks at a time.

Genital herpes

These sores have a tendency to
expand at the penis, round or in
the vagina, at the buttocks, or at
the anus, aleven though they are
able to shape on different regions
of pores and skin.

Herpes also can purpose ache
while urinating and modifications
in vaginal discharge.

The first time someone develops the sores, they will closing 2–6 weeks.

Soon after this preliminary outbreak, signs might also additionally recur frequently. Over time, outbreaks might also additionally arise much less regularly and the signs have a tendency to turn out to be much less extreme.

Primary signs

These arise while someone first develops the contamination.

Alongside sores or blisters, herpes might also additionally purpose:

- ache and itching

- swollen lymph nodes

- a fever

- fatigue and a well-known feeling of being unwell

In maximum instances, the lesions heal with out long-time period scarring.

Recurring signs

Symptoms that reappear are much like the preliminary signs, aleven though they have a tendency to be much less extreme and closing for shorter durations.

Research indicates that round 33% of human beings with oral herpes and 50% of these with genital herpes revel in ordinary signs.

During every recurrence, signs of oral herpes have a tendency to closing 8–10 days, in keeping with the American Sexual Health Association.

Symptoms of a genital herpes recurrence additionally closing 8–10 days, and there could be fewer sores than in the preliminary phase. During a recurrence, someone can by skip on genital herpes for 2–five days.

Causes

When HSV is gift at the pores and skin, it may effortlessly by skip from individual to individual thru touch with the wet pores and skin of the mouth and genitals, which includes the anus.

The virus may unfold thru touch with different regions of the pores and skin and the eyes.

A individual can't agreement HSV through touching an item or a surface, which include a washbasin or towel.

Infection can arise in the following ways:

• having vaginal or anal intercourse with out the use of barrier protection, which include a condom

• sharing intercourse toys

• having some other oral or genital touch with someone who has herpes

The virus is maximum contagious among the time while signs first seem and once they heal. Less commonly, someone can transmit the virus while signs aren't gift.

If a girl with genital herpes has sores at the same time as giving birth, the virus can by skip directly to the baby.

CHAPTER TWO

HSV and HIV

People with genital herpes have a better chance of contracting and passing on HIV, as sores in the pores and skin can facilitate HIV's passing into and out of the body.

HSV-2 will increase the variety of CD4 cells in the genital lining, that may improve the chance of contamination if someone is uncovered to HIV.

Also, human beings with HIV have weakened immune systems, and this will increase the chance of greater extreme complications.

For example, if someone has oral herpes and a weakened immune machine, they will have a better chance of growing keratitis, a form of eye irritation, or encephalitis, irritation of the brain.

If someone has a weakened immune machine and genital herpes, there's, hardly ever, a better chance of growing irritation of the brain, eyes, esophagus, lungs, or liver, in addition to tremendous contamination.

Treatment

There are numerous remedy alternatives for each oral and genital herpes.

Home treatments

The following should assist relieve herpes signs for a few human beings:

• dabbing cornstarch onto the affected area

• squirting water from a bottle onto blisters to ease ache at the same time as urinating

• making use of aloe vera gel to sores

However, no studies suggests that those treatments work.

A individual may also try:

- taking ache remedy medicine, which include acetaminophen or ibuprofen

- bathing in gently salted water or soaking in a heat sitz bath

- making use of petroleum jelly to the affected regions

- carrying unfastened apparel to keep away from irritation

- refraining from sexual interest, inspite of protection, till signs have gone

- making use of a cream or lotion to the urethra earlier than urinating, which include one which consists of lidocaine

Some human beings discover that the use of ice packs assist. Never follow ice without delay to the pores and skin — wrap it in a fabric first.

Medication

No drug can put off the herpes virus. However, a medical doctor might also additionally prescribe an antiviral medicine, which include acyclovir, to save you the virus from multiplying.

Meanwhile, over the counter herpes treatments, that are

regularly creams, can assist control tingling, itching, and ache.

To extensively reduce the period of a virus, begin remedy inside 24 hours of preliminary signs, for example, as quickly because the tingling starts.

If someone makes use of antiviral medicine, signs might also additionally clear up 1–2 days greater fast than in the event that they had used no remedy. Medication may lessen the severity of signs.

If someone has fewer than six recurrences of genital herpes in step with year, a medical doctor might also additionally prescribe an antiviral medicine at every recurrence.

If someone reports recurrences greater frequently, a medical doctor might also additionally suggest taking an antiviral for 6–twelve months at a time.

Taking those medicinal drugs each day for longer durations can extensively lessen the chance of passing herpes to a partner, aleven though it stays a possibility.

Prevention tips

The following techniques can lessen the chance of growing or passing on herpes:

• the use of barrier protection, which include condoms, while having intercourse

• averting intercourse at the same time as signs are gift

• averting kissing and oral intercourse while there's a chilly sore across the mouth

• washing the arms thoroughly, specifically after touching the affected area, at some stage in a virus

Some human beings additionally discover that stress, being tired, illness, pores and skin friction, and sunbathing can cause recurrences of signs.

Identifying and averting those triggers can assist lessen the variety of outbreaks.

CHAPTER THREE

What reasons genital sores in ladies?

Genital sores in ladies have some of ability reasons. The maximum common are sexually transmitted infections (STIs), which includes herpes.

Genital sores because of STIs have a tendency to be painful and itchy. They can seem as one or a couple of sores. These are the maximum common form of genital sores, and that they may be very contagious.

Some bumps at the vulva and in the vagina are painless, at the same time as others can be itchy, painful, or tender. Some might also additionally produce discharge.

It may be very hard to inform the distinction among STIs that purpose genital sores. For this reason, each person with genital sores need to see a medical doctor for correct prognosis and remedy. For a photo manual to assist pick out common STIs, click on here.

This article discusses quite a number STIs which can purpose girl genital sores — which includes herpes, syphilis, and genital warts — in addition to a few non-STI reasons.

Genital herpes

There are some of ability reasons for genital sores.

Genital herpes is a viral STI that reasons outbreaks of blisters at the genitals. In the United States, this common contamination influences greater than 1 in 6 human beings elderly 14–49. It is a common purpose of genital sores.

When a person has a virus of genital herpes, they'll expand one or greater small blister-like lesions across the genitals or rectum. The blisters spoil open and purpose painful genital sores. The sores commonly take every week or greater to solve.

Most human beings with genital herpes don't have any signs or moderate signs, so maximum human beings do now no longer realize that they've it. This makes it smooth to transmit from individual to individual.

Genital herpes isn't always presently curable, however the variety of outbreaks has a tendency to lessen over time. People can shorten outbreaks the use of medicinal drugs, and a few capsules can substantially lessen the chance of transmitting the virus to sexual partners.

Syphilis

Syphilis is some other STI, this time characterized through one or greater painless ulcers known as chancres. They are commonly corporation and spherical.

Syphilis is due to micro organism called Treponema pallidum. Chancres have a tendency to seem 10–ninety days after publicity to the micro organism.

The ulcers usually clear up inside three–6 weeks. However, with out remedy, syphilis might also additionally purpose severe complications.

A route of intravenous penicillin G can deal with syphilis. After remedy, someone might also additionally want to go through some other check to ensure that the contamination has cleared up.

Chancroid

Chancroid is an STI characterized through painful genital ulcers and painful, swollen lymph glands in the groin area. It is due to micro organism known as Haemophilus ducreyi.

Chancroid lesions start off as small, pink bumps and fast change into pustules, or acne that include pus. These pustules burst to turn out to be very painful ulcers. The ulcers might also additionally bleed effortlessly.

Without remedy, the ulcers might also additionally closing for 1–three months.

It might also additionally take four–10 days after sexual touch to expand chancroid, aleven though it may take so long as 35 days.

Once remedy has begun, signs have a tendency to enhance inside three days, and the contamination commonly clears up inside 7 days. Large ulcers might also additionally want round 2 weeks to heal.

CHAPTER FOUR

Molluscum contagiosum

Molluscum contagiosum is a contagious pores and skin contamination that reasons small lesions or bumps to expand at the thighs, buttocks, groin, and decrease abdomen.

The lesions also can seem at the genitals and across the anus and might change into large sores that turn out to be itchy or tender. They may be flesh colored, gray-white, yellow, or pink.

The lesions might also additionally closing from 2 weeks to four years.

Most lesions heal naturally, aleven though they will come back. Doctors can cast off them to save you them from spreading to others.

Granuloma inguinale

Granuloma inguinale is an STI that reasons deep pink ulcers that bleed. However, those ulcers have a tendency to be painless. The contamination is due to micro organism known as Klebsiella granulomatis.

People can deal with this contamination the use of antibiotics, aleven though it can go back 6–18 months later.

Non-STI reasons

Although maximum genital sores arise because of STIs, there are numerous ability non-STI reasons. In very uncommon instances, genital sores might also additionally expand because of cancer, or they will be innocent cysts that a medical doctor can cast off.

Some different non-STI reasons of girl genital sores include:

Non-sexually received genital ulceration

Non-sexually received genital ulceration (NSAGU) is a situation that reasons painful ulcers to expand across the genitals. Recurrent instances are greater common in ladies than males.

The ulcers can seem as unmarried or a couple of shallow, spherical sores. In ladies, they are able to seem constantly or infrequently, or they will seem regularly, which include earlier than menstruation every month.

Doctors do now no longer realize the precise purpose of NSAGU, however it seems to be connected with immune machine characteristic and underlying fitness conditions, which include celiac disease or Crohn's disorder.

Hidradenitis suppurativa

Hidradenitis suppurativa is a persistent situation that reasons pus stuffed bumps, difficult bumps, or open wounds that don't drain. These bumps and wounds can seem on and beneath the pores and skin.

The bumps have a tendency to arise in regions wherein the pores and skin rubs together, which include the groin and armpits. They may be huge and painful.

Psoriasis

Psoriasis is a persistent pores and skin situation due to an overgrowth of pores and skin cells. There are numerous kinds of psoriasis, and a few can purpose sores at the pores and skin.

Pustular psoriasis, for example, reasons white, pus stuffed blisters which could burst and turn out to be open sores. When the blisters disappear, the pores and skin might also additionally turn out to be scaly.

Guttate psoriasis, on the alternative hand, reasons small dot-like lesions throughout the pores and skin.

Behcet's disorder

Behcet's disorder is a unprecedented inflammatory situation that reasons ulcers at the mouth and genitals, pores and skin lesions, and eye abnormalities.

The ulcers are commonly spherical or oval with reddish borders. In ladies, they have a tendency to have an effect on the vulva. They commonly heal inside some days, however they are able to seem and recur spontaneously.

Healthcare specialists do now no longer realize the purpose of

Behcet's disorder, however it's far possibly connected with genetics.

Other reasons

Other elements also can purpose genital sores, which includes bodily or sexual trauma.

Diagnosis

Because there are lots of ability reasons of girl genital sores, it's far vital to go to a medical doctor for a prognosis as quickly as possible. This will make sure that someone gets the proper remedy.

To decide the purpose of the sores, a medical doctor will perform a bodily exam. They may want to carry out different tests, which include taking blood samples or a swab from the affected area.

How to save you STIs

Using barrier methods, which include condoms, at some stage in sexual interest is the best manner to save you STIs. Condoms are to be had to buy over the counter.

To save you transmitting STIs which include herpes and syphilis to a sexual partner, someone need to now no longer have interaction in any sexual touch at some stage in a virus of this type of conditions. They need to chorus from intercourse till the signs have subsided.

Outlook

Most reasons of genital sores are effortlessly treatable the use of medicinal drugs. When a bacterium reasons the sores, a quick route of antibiotics will commonly solve the contamination.

Some conditions, which include herpes, are lifelong, and those will revel in breakouts from time to time. If a person starts to revel in breakouts, they need to see their medical doctor.

It is vital to apprehend what's inflicting the hassle to realize a way to deal with it. A individual need to consequently see a medical doctor at the primary signal of a genital sore.

THE END

www.ingramcontent.com/pod-product-compliance
Lightning Source LLC
Chambersburg PA
CBHW070745260726
48660CB00007B/2993